WALKING: WALK 10,000 STEPS PER DAY PLAN

BEST EXERCISE TO LOSE WEIGHT AND GET FIT AT ANY AGE AND CURRENT FITNESS LEVEL

I0435434

DAVID BARRAZA

www.davidbarrazanaturalhealth.com

TABLE OF CONTENTS:

DEDICATION

This book is dedicated to any health conscious person out there, and anybody looking to improve their body and mind through a healthier lifestyle. Walking is such a low impact exercise that it can be practiced by almost anybody regardless of age, weight or current fitness level.

I'm writing this dedication on January 1, 2016, a perfect time to commit to an exercise program and setup new health goals for the New Year. Most people make New Year's Resolutions. Almost always at the top of the list is to eat healthier and get started on some type of exercise or fitness program.

I sincerely wish you find this book helpful on making walking a daily habit in your life. Like anything worth having in life, it will take dedication, time and an honest commitment. A walking program aiming at 10,000 steps per day may seem like a long shot, but I promise you it can be rather fun and enjoyable if you have the right mindset and motivation.

Let's get walking.

INTRODUCTION

My experience with walking is that in addition to its health benefits, it can also be very enjoyable and relaxing. Some of the happiest moments of my life have been while I'm doing long walks and I let go of all worries in my mind and just enjoy the surroundings. You don't always get every walk to be so fulfilling and enjoyable, but if you practice walking long enough, you'll get a good number of great walks that will motivate you to make walking a daily habit.

After you make a habit of walking daily (or at least 4-5 times a week), it doesn't take long before you'll start seeing gradual but steady benefits. If you stick to it, you'll start loving it so much you won't ever want to quit walking. You soon will see many benefits like an improved mood, feeling energized, a better sleep, weight loss, improved digestion and overall better health.

In addition to burning calories and other health benefits walking will give you an overall "feel-good" sensation. You may have heard of Endorphins, which are chemicals produced by your body under stimulus like certain foods, sex or exercise. Even though endorphins are produced mainly during intense exercise like a heavy weight training session or long runs, I've found you may get some of this same feeling if your walks go for around 45 minutes or longer.

I'm a long distance runner (I run half marathons and marathons), and I get to feel the runners-high, which is that euphoric sensation you feel after a long or intense run. Even so, I'm still doing long walks rather frequently to give my legs a break from running and because long walks can actually be more relaxing than my runs. Long walks have a lower impact in my body, therefore less likely I'll get injured. Plus, some of the benefits of running can be replicated with long walks with almost none of the possible side effects of running like inflammation, knee and hip pain, blisters, etc.

In this book I will cover the different aspects of a successful walking plan. I'll discuss with you about motivation, walking gear, planning of your walks, where to walk and so forth. I will layout step by step all you need to know to get to walk up to 10,000 per day, 5-6 times a week and get all the physical and mental benefits of walking. If you wish and feel like walking more than the 10,000 per day, you're welcome to do so, as long as your body can adapt to it and you can get additional benefits from it.

I wish you a healthy and happy life with enjoyable long walks!

CHAPTER 1:
ARE YOU HAPPY WITH YOUR CURRENT WEIGHT, HEALTH AND FITNESS LEVEL?

If you are reading this book, chances are you are not happy with your current health, weight or fitness level. Even if you are not unhappy, you may still be considering ways to improve your health, weight, fitness level and/or overall wellbeing.

Assessing your current weight and overall health:

How much do you weigh and what should your ideal weight be?

Most people gain weight as they age, it seems like is inevitable and the normal thing to happen. I actually don't agree with this. After going to College and getting into the normal 9 to 5 type of schedule routine, with all kind of odd schedules and jobs, the past few years after dedicating myself seriously into running and working out, I'm almost as slim as in my High School years. I definitely think life style is the main reason people get out of shape as they age. Aging does seem to slow down your metabolism, how soon you recover from working out and illnesses but in a lesser degree compared to lifestyle.

You may have a good idea about how close (or not) you are to your ideal body weight just by looking yourself at the mirror, or if you are using a scale from time to time. It's a good idea though to take a look at some matrixes regarding the recommended weight for adults over 20.

The US government recommends an ideal weight range based on your height. This ideal weight range is called the BMI (Body Mass Index). The range is rather wide and my personal experience with weight is that you should aim for the lower range of your BMI. You can use a simple calculator of your BMI by going to the Centers for Disease Control and Prevention's (CDC) website at http://www.cdc.gov/healthyweight/assessing/, URL valid as of January 2, 2016. Once you land on the page, you want to click on the left side on the Adult BMI Calculator. You simply enter your height and weight and click on the Calculate button. You will get a figure along an assessment of your weight. The BMI will range from below 18.5 to 30.0 and above, it will also have a corresponding weight status ranging from Underweight to Obese. The BMI reading also shows you additional details of your normal weight range depending on your height. Example: a 5'10" male weights 165 Lbs., it has a reading of a 23.7 BMI. This BMI falls under the Normal weight status. A normal BMI range is considered to be between 18.5 and 24.9 according to the CDC.

As I mentioned before the BMI should be used as a general guideline and not as the only source to calculate your ideal recommended weight. Some of the new scales in the market also give you a Fat Mass percentage reading. This is different than the BMI. The Fat Mass % is simply a calculation of your fat mass in relation to your overall weight. Using the same example of the 165 Lbs. and 5'10" male, he may have a reading of around 8-15% fat mass. For this guy, that percentage definitely will be on the lean side and you will be able to see a decent set of abs. To give you an idea, if you ever seen those super lean and rather freaky looking professional bodybuilders on TV, on the internet or on magazines, they normally have a 5% or lower fat mass percentage when they look like that. Even for super competitive athletes, a 5% or lower fat mass reading is not considered healthy if maintained for long periods of time (say, more than 2-3 weeks) at a time. To get to such a low percentage of fat mass, normally a very strict diet is followed for a few weeks, along with multiple cardio sessions (in some cases more than one session per day).

If you are reading this book, likely you are not a professional athlete and you shouldn't aim to have a fat mass under 5%. First of all because of the strict diet this involves, the intense cardio sessions and lastly because your immune system will weaken dramatically, not to mention your mood swings will get very wild.

If you don't already own a scale, consider investing in one. There are many out there for all budgets and personal preferences and needs. The traditional scales like the ones you find at your Doctor's office, are the most reliable but also the ones that give you the least amount of data. You get your weight (and often your height is measured at the same time), and that's about it.

You can get your weight taken for free at the Doctor's office, at the mall for 25 cents or if you are a member of gym or health club some will have scales for you to use. I definitely have found helpful investing in a scale. The free options mentioned before may not be available or not as often as you need them to track your weight frequently. Out of all the brands out there, I personally like the *Withings* brand. The scale I bought is a *smart scale* that will measure your weight, your body fat percentage and your heart rate and even temperature and weather conditions. You can find this scale for around $140 US Dollars at some higher- end sports stores or online retailers such as

Amazon. I considered buying this scale an investment in my health for years to come. Consider your budget and needs when investing in a scale. Weigh yourself once a week for best results and to keep you motivated.

How good is your health right now? There are some indicators you can use to assess your health. The main ones are the obvious you get from your doctor like your weight, blood pleasure and lack of disease/s. Other indicators as important, but not as obvious would be your overall wellbeing in regards to how good you feel on a regular basis, how productive you are at work, how fulfilling your personal and/or family relationships are and how happy and positive you feel day in and day out.

Blood Pressure:

I already mentioned the topic on weight. Let's talk briefly about blood pressure now. Your Doctor or Medical Professional is the best one to measure your blood pleasure, but you can also buy some over the counter devices at a very affordable price that do this at your local pharmacy. I found an inexpensive watch at my local Walmart that measures your blood pleasure after your press your finger at a sensor reader for a few seconds. This watch also is useful to do my step counting when I go out for my walks among other useful things. I personally don't consider as important measuring you blood pleasure as often as weighing yourself, unless you have a health condition that requires you to do so.

Blood pressure has two readings: A 'top number' or Systolic and a 'bottom number' or Diastolic. Not that you really need to know, but the blood pressure readings are given in *mm Hg* (millimeters of mercury). The Mayo Clinic staff has established four blood pressure categories. This blood pressure chart can help you figure out if your blood pressure is at a healthy level or if you'll need to take some steps to improve your numbers:

http://www.mayoclinic.org/diseases-conditions/high-blood-pressure/in-depth/blood-pressure/art-20050982

If you have **Systolic/Top #:** Below 120, **Diastolic/bottom:** And below 80**, Your Category:** Normal blood pressure, **What to do:** Maintain or adopt a healthy lifestyle.

If you have **Systolic/Top #:** Between 120-139, **Diastolic/bottom:** Or between 80-99**, Your Category:** Prehypertension, **What to do:** Maintain or adopt a healthy lifestyle.

If you have **Systolic/Top #:** Between 140-159, **Diastolic/bottom:** Or between 90-99**, Your Category:** Stage 1 hypertension, **What to do:** Maintain or adopt a healthy lifestyle. If your blood pressure goal isn't reached in about a month, talk to your doctor about taking one or more medications.

If you have **Systolic/Top #:** 160 or higher, **Diastolic/bottom:** Or 100 or higher**, Your Category:** Stage 2 hypertension, **What to do:** Maintain or adopt a healthy lifestyle. Talk to your doctor about taking more than one medication.

*Check the provided URL (website address) for more details and a better understanding of the blood pressure readings.

I recently noticed while driving by my neighborhood, that some pharmacies offer free health evaluations. These normally consist of a general health checkup for free. Take advantage of this option if is available to you.

How is your fitness level right now?

There are some non-medical/formal ways to have an idea of your current fitness level. Use these as general guidelines as they are not medical but rather useful common sense advises:

Short 5-10 minutes walks: Do you feel exhausted after very short walks? If you have this feeling after 10 or less minutes of a moderate pace (one you can keep while holding a conversation), chances are you fitness level is not good.

Try walking up a set of stairs: If climbing up a 1 or 2 story set of stairs gets you grasping for air, it definitely tells you your fitness can use some improvement.

House or physical work shores: If doing the day to day house or work shores like washing dishes (by hand), doing laundry, vacuuming, mowing the lawn and you get very tired or exhausted after 10 minutes or less, you need to improve your fitness.

Overall energy level: If your energy level during work or any activity (not physically intense) is rather low, and your mood is rather cranky, this can also be an indicator of a poor fitness level and/or overall poor health.

Overall happiness and family or personal relationships:

Do you find yourself having difficulty to get along with people? Do you get easily frustrated when talking or interacting with people around you? If you answered yes to any of these questions, first of all find out if this happens most of the time or is just from time to time or rather rare. Try to find out if this is due to any specific event like downsizing of your company, bigger work load, etc. If you can't find any specific good reason, check how is your sleep, how well are you eating and if you have any regular exercise program going on, otherwise poor overall fitness (and eventually poor health) may cause to have you in a bad mood with low tolerance to frustration.

How is your productivity at work, business or at home? Have you noticed you are unable to complete your tasks at work, your business or at home? If so, think of any specific trigger you may have noticed recently like a family event, you've gotten a serious illness recently, financial stress, etc. If you cannot think of any of the previous reasons, think if you've noticed being less productive as a slow gradual process for weeks, months or years. If the second scenario is what you can tell is happening, consider this being related to a gradual process of poor eating and exercise habits.

CHAPTER 2
WHY WALKING?

Walking is such a natural and uncomplicated exercise that if may be look down upon when compared to any other more intense or complicated exercise or sport. If may not be even seen as exercise but rather a natural way to get from point A to point B for a short distance.

As a natural process of the human being development, most babies learn to walk between 9-12 months, but it's perfectly normal to take longer than that. After that walking will be used to move around and explore the surroundings.

Natural weight loss and weight control by walking:

I remember growing up in a village until I was 7 when we move to a small city. In this village most people didn't have a car. The economy was based mostly on agriculture a cattle. One thing I remember is most people will walk to the field to grow corn or beans or vegetables and to take care of their cattle. Some will ride their horses or donkeys and a few others will drive their trucks. In general most people from small kids to adults will do a good amount of walking every day.

When my family moved to the city, most people will still do a good deal of walking as the city was rather small. Going to work or school was only a few blocks away. Eventually as our family moved around _I noticed when I lived in communities where people_ *would mostly drive to move around, people were heavier* and seemed to also have more problems with diseases associated with being overweight like diabetes, high blood pressure, etc.

Even though walking or the lack thereof is not the only factor that determines your body weight, it seems to be an important one. In most cities, the kids take the bus to school and teenagers and young adults either also take the bus, have someone give them a lift and some that live closer to school or college will walk. The same thing applies when commuting to and from work.

I remember when I was younger and going to college and didn't have a car, taking the bus to work and school will still make me walk some. Once I had a car, it was convenient and fast, but I noticed right away after just a few months I started gaining a bit of weight until I started working out and was able to shed the few pounds I've gained.

Mood booster and psychological benefits of walking:

In my books introduction, I already mentioned the benefits of walking due to the production of endorphins (usually during the longer walks of over 45 minutes). Consider also the use of a daily walking routine as a way to relax and unplug from your daily routing of work and occupations. Be it with a friend or by yourself walking is a great way to reduce your stress and worries that otherwise may keep you up all night or worse even, push you into unhealthy habits of drinking, drugs or binge eating among others if the level of stress because unbearable

How many calories do you burn when you walk?

Depending on your weight and how fast you walk the calories burned will vary. Data from the US Government estimates a 5'10", 154 Lb. male burns approximately 280 calories/hour at a 3.5 mph (miles per hour) pace. This is considered a moderately fast pace, but not a fast walking pace. These calories include both the calories used by the activity and the calories used for the normal body functioning during the activity time. In other words, we consume calories even when we are sitting down or even sleeping (at a very low rate of course). Those who weigh more will burn more calories and those who weigh less will burn fewer calories.

CHAPTER 3
WHAT DO YOU NEED TO START A WALKING PROGRAM?

Gadgets/Devices to count steps and calories burned during your walk:

Obviously you can use the general guideline listed at the end of the previous chapter as a free calories burned counter during your walks. That will be the bare minimum next to not counting your calories at all. Some people may find counting calories cumbersome, and may prefer just to count your walk time wise, it that's you, go for it if you feel it may work for you.

My experience is that you get best results when you measure and get an actual figure of your calories burned. There are so many and inexpensive or free ways to do it. Chances are you own a cell phone that _comes already with_ some sort of _fitness app_ that can measure your walking calories after it has the reading of your time and steps taken, this may involve turning on GPS, which most phones come equipped with nowadays. Be aware of possible data rates applicable on your cell phone plan. You can also download a free app from Google Play, App Store or corresponding platform depending on your phone.

My preferred method is to invest in a fitness gadget. Find out online (YouTube product reviews is probably the best way), or Google for Fitness Trackers or ask your friends and get what best fits your budget and preferences. The products I like and I've used myself are Fitbit, Jawbone and Bodymedia (now part of Jawbone) among some other free apps. The best thing about these wearables is that you can see your progress live when connected to your smartphone app (usually via Bluetooth). You can preset your 10,000 steps daily goal and track your progress during the day. I found that the apps that are linked to your fitness gadget will also come with additional useful features like calorie intake tracker, overall calories burned, etc. This gives an advantage to the free step counting stand-alone apps.

And lastly, you can invest in a GPS or pedometer enabled watch. These may track steps, distance and calories burned. You'll find also all kind of product for all budgets and preferences. I'm personally a big fan of Garmin GPS enabled fitness device. It's by far the brand that I've found gives you the most data. I use it mainly because it's my preferred way to track my runs as well. Again, depending on your goals, budgets and personal preferences you may decide what device to use or if you prefer to not invest on any product and you track your progress solely with how you feel and look.

Walking sneakers or shoes: Walking does not need any pricey or fancy pair of shoes or sneakers. You can do you daily walking routine in your existing worn out sneaker or shoes. The most important thing is for them to be comfortable. Have in mind if you're going to be walking more than you currently do, you may have to replace them soon.

Other than shoes being comfortable, consider if they'd need to be washed often. My experience with long walks is that sneakers are typically more comfortable than shoes. Consider getting a pair of comfortable, low to the ground (thin sole) pair of sneakers if you don't already own a pair. The lower to the ground your walking shoes or sneakers are, the more natural your walking will be. To get started wear whatever you already have and as you make walking a daily habit, your feet may 'start asking you' for a pair of sneakers more comfortable, with more support if you find yourself long walks make your feet hurt.

On a side note, if you live close to the ocean, a great drill is to walk barefoot from time to time. This makes your toes and feet stronger and improves your walking form. An alternate option is to walk barefoot on grass at the park, or just practice being barefoot from time to time at your front or back yard and inside your home. You will notice over time walking becomes more natural. After all we weren't born wearing shoes.

Wear a pair of comfortable synthetic socks:

Long walks are not quite like running, but if you find yourself prone to blistering or your feet tend to get rather sweaty during your walks, a good pair of synthetic (not cotton) socks is a good investment. Synthetic fabric in general is more breathable than cotton, it can last longer and price wise there's not a big difference. Cotton socks can be warmer, therefore you may want to stick to them for the warmer summer months or if you really like the extra cushioning they give you.

Use Vaseline or similar lubricant if you blister easily:

Walking is usually an exercise that does not cause irritation or blisters. But if you have sensitive skin, or have a medical condition that may cause poor circulation to your feet (like diabetes or some skin condition), using Vaseline or another lubricant may be useful. This should be applied around the areas where you may have some friction like your heels, the inner and outer side 'the ball of your feet" (wider area in front of your foot arch). Lubricant should also be applied around your toes and in between them.

Consider baby powder if your feet get too sweaty:

If blisters are not your problem, but your feet get too sweaty, baby power is a good option you may want to consider. Some people walk or run in a nice breathable pair of sneakers and don't need to worry about wearing socks, applying Vaseline/lubricant or baby power. It's worth trying it if you're curious.

CHAPTER 4
10,000 STEPS PER DAY WALKING PLAN

If you've made it reading up to this chapter of the book, I congratulate you and appreciate your patience. I have the feeling you are really serious about the 10,000 steps per day walking plan. This is definitely the most exciting part of the book for me. Let's get down to layout the plan, are you ready?

Step 1: Make a serious commitment to walk 10,000 steps every day:

Purchasing this book was the first and most important step. You may be already walking on your own, or may be thinking walking doesn't need a plan and you can just go out and start walking on your own. Even though this can be true, I found out with my experience with running marathons that having a plan and commitment increases the chances of succeeding. Before I got committed to running my fist Half Marathon and eventually my first full Marathon, I would just go out to the park and run for 30-45 minutes on the weekends or whenever I had the time or was in the mood. Even though this was better than nothing, I knew I needed a plan to be able to run a Marathon at a decent pace someday.

Once I made the commitment to run my first Half Marathon, I took action: First I went to the running store, got my running assessment done, bought my recommended pair of running shoes, my GPS running gadget and downloaded a running plan for a Half Marathon distance. Long story short, 4 months after I started my running plan, I finished my first Half Marathon ever, and 5 months after that my very first every full Marathon (9 months after starting running). I could've done both distances sooner, but I was rather ambitious and wanted to run decent times on both races... and I did.

All I want to say with this pep talk is... you need to be committed to succeed to accomplish your goal to walk 10,000 steps per day. On the previous chapters I talked about some investment regarding a pair of sneakers, a smart watch/gadget or free app to track your progress and keep you motivated and also some additional things to consider like synthetic socks and lubricants or baby powder. If you decided you don't need to invest on anything but still feel committed to this program, you are ready for step 2 of this program.

Step 2: Setup a schedule for your daily walks:

This is a very important step. The best time for your daily walks will depend on your work, school or whatever daily commitments or activities you have going on.

For the typical 9-5 work schedule, you have some flexibility to do your walks before or after work. If you have kids and need to get them ready to school, child care, etc. before you go to work, you'll have to get up rather early to get in your daily walk. Consider doing part of your daily walk/s early in the morning and the rest after work or school.

Sticking to a schedule is important as a discipline, but be flexible as needed. The most important thing is to walk 10,000 steps (or more) per day, not necessarily doing your walks at the exact same time every day. Also use your body's energy level during the day to determine what time may be best for your walks. A common belief is that the best time to do any type of workout is in the morning, if it works for you do it, otherwise chose a time that fits you best.

Step 3: Where to Walk? Choose at least 2 or 3 places or routes to walk:

Choosing a place is to do you daily walks is important for different reasons:

It needs to be a place you can easily get to every day or most days. To be able to get all your walks done every day, the place has to be accessible, hopefully not too far from home or in the way to or from work. If you doing mind driving a few minutes, I don't recommend more than 10 to get to the park, trail or streets you want to do you walks on. It doesn't make sense choosing a great place with great views, clean air, etc. if you know it won't be easy to get there every day to do your walks.

Chose a place you like and motivates you to do your walks. It can be your neighborhood, the park nearby, walking around a mall, etc. Pick out place you enjoy seeing while you walk, this will motivate you to stick with your walking daily routine. I see it difficult walking around a place I don't like on a regular basis. Chose something you like based on your personal preferences like nature, flat/hilly roads, with traffic of people, etc.

Find a place that is safe. It's an obvious recommendation but if you chose a place you're not familiar with, find out first if is safe to be there, ask your friends or family or go online and find out as much as you can about the neighborhood or location. The last feeling you want to have when walking is fear or how soon you have to leave the place because is not safe to be there.

It's a good idea to have at least two or three places to walk. Even if you have a favorite spot to walk, you may eventually find yourself bored of seeing the same streets, same homes or buildings. Consider choosing a different path for your daily walks even if is around the same area or neighborhood. You'd be surprised how with simply changes like taking the street next to the one you always take, walking at a park instead of the neighborhood, etc. feels like an entire different experience during your walk.

Step 4: Walking pace: How long will it take you to walk 10,000 steps?

On average, 2000 steps is about a mile, so walking 10,000 steps means walking about 5 miles. This may seem like a lot, but consider the 10,000 steps as the total number steps you take on a given day, not only during you actual *walking workout.* This is why it would be so useful to have a way to track your steps at all times during the day. Once again, consider one of the options offered on Chapter 3 of this book. I find it hard to track all the steps you will take during the day if you just use your own mental calculation.

Most of us walk briskly at about 3.5 miles per hour, which takes about 17 minutes per mile or about 85 minutes for 5 miles. That translates into 1 hour and 25 minutes for your 10,000 steps. Have in mind that depending on your work and daily activities, you may only have to walk part of the remaining steps in your walking session to get to your 10,000 steps in one day. I for example, walk between 4,000 and 5,000 on a regular day without including my actual walking or running workouts. These steps are just from walking to my car, I take the stairways whenever I can instead of the elevator (4 stories up in the morning and then 4 stories down in the afternoon), a couple of trips to the break room and rest room during the day and the steps count add up. You can do a few tricks to walk more like parking the farthest possible and safe from your office or work place, use the stairs instead of the elevator, walk instead of driving to do some errands like trips to the pharmacy, convenience store, etc.

If you on the other hand have a rather sedentary type of job, you'll definitely have to spend more time doing the actual walking session.

Step 5: Walking Technique: I recommend a brisk pace for better results and to hopefully save you some time during your daily walks. But be aware of your current weight and fitness level and walk at a pace that is comfortable and won't force your body to go faster that it can. As you stick to your plan, your fitness will improve and you'll be able to walk faster and longer.

As for your walking technique, use the following recommendations as a useful guide: Look forward not to the ground, move your shoulders naturally, keep your chin parallel to the ground, keep your back straight not arched forward or backward, stomach tighten gently, swing your arms freely with elbows slightly bent, walk smoothly rolling your feet from feet from heel to toe.

Let your body adjust to this recommended technique, but also try to make it feel natural. Practicing a good walking technique should not leave you exhausted after a few minutes nor should it make your body feel oddly uncomfortable. I'm noticed that when you try walking faster, that forces your body to be more efficient, use that as a good indicator or how a good technique should feel and look like. If needed, alternate periods of 5-15 minutes of fast walking with up to 30 minutes of a comfortable walking pace, which is a pace you can keep a conversation going one without heavy breathing between full sentences.

Step 6: Benefits of splitting up your daily walk into 2 or more sessions:

Schedule and weather: If you find yourself unable to do all 10,000 steps in a single session, try doing one morning session and one late afternoon/night session. The steps you do in each session will depend on your own schedule and/or preference. In the winter I prefer to do all or most of my walks in the late afternoon or early at night since I start work early. Getting up at 3 or 4 a.m. when is super dark and cold wouldn't be practical.

Fitness level: If you feel like walking for an hour and 25 minutes straight is not something you may be able to do when you start your walking program, splitting up your 10,000 per day in 2 or more sessions also makes perfect sense. This will also keep you from getting extremely tired or possibly injuring yourself by forcing your body beyond what it's physically ready for.

Additional stress relief: This will be especially useful if you have a job or activity that is rather stressful. Doing part of your walking in the morning will have you fresher when you start work and the second session will help you with blowing off some steam and relax after a long stressful day and prepare you for a deep restful sleep.

It keeps your mind fresh from the routine: Walking at different times of the day will add variety to your daily walks. If you have an open mind, you'd be surprised how different it feels walking early in the morning instead of noon or night. It's not only the weather different, but also the activity level happening at different times of day. For quiet relaxing walks you may want to choose early mornings or late night walks, whereas for energetic and fast walks (weather permitting), a good time may be in in the afternoon or early nights. If you definitely prefer to walk with a friend, your time choices will depend on your friend's schedule too, but if it helps you keeping motivated, go for it. If you have a flexible schedule, chose a time of the day that better suits your mood and level or energy and location preference.

Step 7: Keep a daily, weekly and monthly log of your steps taken:

Your chances of succeeding on your goal will increase dramatically if you use a method to track your daily walking sessions and steps taken. At the beginning of Chapter 3 I gave you different options available to track your steps and sessions in general. I mentioned the convenience of using a wearable device that tracks your steps along other useful data.

If you are in a budget, you can still get things done with some creativity. I only see this option reasonably possible to count your walking session, not practical at all if you're planning on counting the 'extra' steps you take during your normal daily activities. The *extreme low budget* option would be to manually count your steps (I know it sound crazy and boring), but it works if you really want to go in this route. People may start calling you the step counter or other not so kind names. As you fine tune your walk sessions, you may be able to calculate approximately the number of steps from point to point on whatever route you've chosen. Let's say it takes you 45 minutes to do 2 laps at your local park, which is slightly over half of the 85 minutes it would normally take to walk 10,000 steps at a brisk pace. If you do around 4 laps instead of 2, you'd have completed your goal for the day. Another option is to time your walks. Once you walk for 85 minutes total for the day at a brisk pace you'd accomplish your daily goal for total steps. This is not my preferred method, but it works if you really want to get it done without investing on any tracking device. You will have to be very honest while tracking yourself your steps or distance divided by the time to calculate the steps taken.

If you decided to go with the extreme low budget option, once you have determined the steps taken for that day, you'll log the daily count on journal or notepad. Will be best if you have access to a spreadsheet software program like Microsoft Excel or similar where you can easily design a log table where you log in the steps count for each day. Then you can use the built in software to track your averages weekly, monthly and even yearly if you make the commitment of walking for a year or more as a habit. The information below was already mentioned on Chapter 3, but now it gives additional information and comparisons.

The best free tracking option I've found is to use a cell phone app. Most phones come already with some health or fitness app the lets you do your step tracking. Otherwise, you can download a step tracking or health app from the Google Play Store, the App Store or Windows version equivalent depending on the platform and maker of your phone. You'll just have to search for fitness tracker, step counter or health as the keywords to find the app. The reviews are useful with screenshots or descriptions to find what you may be looking for. This solution does all the tracking for you without any investment, as long as you have a cell phone that is GPS enabled.

If you were to invest in device to track your walk sessions, they usually come already with the software to track your progress. I highly recommend this as the best option as it takes all the guess work and hassle out the picture. The advantages of these devices, also called wearables are that most of them you don't even notice you're wearing them, they wear like a regular watch and many of them are even smaller and discrete. Some have a screen or small display to show your data, but almost all of them (if they come with Bluetooth capabilities) will connect to your smartphone where you'll have a more detailed display of the data and additional features. I find very motivating seeing my progress as I walk, or at the end of the day when my app shows I have completed my goals. Additional features I like from the wearables are sleep tracking, calorie burned count, heart rate, workouts, etc. The features available will vary depending on brand and price. Getting a wearable/fitness tracker makes more sense if you see it as an investment and you are committed to your health in the long run.

CHAPTER 5
MEASURING RESULTS

In the previous chapters I mentioned the convenience of having a systemic way of tracking your daily walks. If you still haven't decided if you'd invest in a fitness tracker, another gadget or simply go by time or manually logging in your daily walks, I once more encourage you to invest in a tracker that suits your budget and preference.

Walking in general should be seeing as something you enjoy. I'd hate that you stop your goal of walking 10,000 steps per day simply because you hate logging in your walks every day. Therefore my insistence with having a way to track this automatically for you and keep your walking experience as something you look forward to every day.

How do I measure my progress?

Weight loss:

 If losing weight was one of the reasons to start a daily walking plan, you should see your weight starting to drop within a few days. Depending on how aggressive and dedicated you want to be with your weight loss, you may also want to start tracking your food intake. An easy plan that works for me is to have a daily deficit of 500 calories. With this plan, you can lose 1 Lb. per week. If you want to be more aggressive, simply adjust this formula to your liking. Say you prefer to lose 2 Lbs. per week, and then you will need a daily calorie deficit of 1000 calories. If you chose a gadget to track your daily walks, most of them will also measure how many calories you burn during the walk and the entire day (even while you're sleeping). The one thing you'll still have to do is to manually log in your food intake. For this there are multiple Apps for your smartphone or you can do this online on your regular computer, tablet or iPad. I've found myfitnesspal (now owned by Under Armor) to be the most complete app to track your food intake, it also allows to manually enter your workouts (like walking) and it even has some great weight loss plans you can use for free. Try to weigh in yourself at least once a week for best results and keep yourself motivated. You have no idea how good it feels when you see the scale giving you a lighter weight every week. Don't be discouraged if you don't lose weight every single week, or if you see some weeks even gain some weight. Be honest and analyze your diet and how well are you sticking to your walking plan if that happens.

Improved health and fitness level:

After a few days of consistent walking, you should start noticing your walks may become easier to complete and you may not get as tired after your walks. You may be able to complete the whole 10,000 steps in one single session in at least in some of your walks. Also make sure you measure your hearth rate, your blood pressure as often as possible. If you have a device that helps talking these readings, that'd be great, if not you next visit to your Doctor should see some improvements. If you don't have a regular yearly appointment with a Doctor, consider getting an appointment in around 3 months after you start and stick to your walking program.

Increased energy levels and general wellness:

These are the results I personally care the most about. The weight loss and improvement fitness will make you feel good as a natural consequence. You should also see some improvement on your sleep, with a deeper sleep during the night and more refreshed and energized feeling during the day. Be aware of making gradual progress in all areas such as your level of exercise (walking plan), your calorie intake and getting enough sleep every night. You may need to adjust as you go through this plan, some adjustments may include more if you realize you're feeling tired and are not eating enough to get all your daily calorie needs to get all your activities done. And be aware that even if you are very overweight, losing weight too fast is not the healthiest option in the long run. Losing more than 3 pounds a week may not be recommended unless you are under a Doctor's supervision.

Less cravings or desire to eat unhealthy food:

This 'health indicator' is real, very real, but you'd have to pay attention to everything you're doing health-wise to find out the reason of less or more cravings towards unhealthy food like sugary, processed, salty or greasy food.

As a rule of thumb, if you're eating enough and healthy natural food, the less likely you are to have food cravings.

As an example, I was able to quit coffee and a need for a sugar boost in the morning by drinking a green leafy veggies and banana every morning before work. I'd get a bit earlier, make the smoothie and drink it while I was getting ready to work. After a only 1-2 weeks I had no cravings for coffee, candy or soda in the morning. I also of course made an effort to get enough sleep at night as that was also a reason why I'd drink coffee in the morning to make me feel awake. Again, healthy changes on habits do make a change, and this can happen fairly quickly.

CHAPTER 6
BEYOND 10,000 STEPS PER DAY

I consider most people will be able to notice health changes within 3-6 months. By this I mean you are the 'standard' person with some extra pounds, not especially overweight but someone that can make some changes towards a healthier lifestyle.

If you are super dedicated towards the 10,000 steps per day plan, along with a healthier way of eating and getting enough sleep at night, you may see results in as little as a few days. The same way applies if you are slow on making changes and may skip your daily walks often. If may take you more than 3 months to see any benefits, you may even not see any noticeable changes if you don't make a compromise to this walking plan and a healthier lifestyle. You are the only one than can determine if this is going to work for you.

What to do if you've succeeded on your 10,000 steps per day and want new challenges?

If you're reading this last chapter of my book, I really hope that means either you were too interested on getting as much useful information as possible or, you are revisiting this chapter after you've reached your goal of 10,000 steps per day, have seen health and fitness improvements and you are looking for new challenges. Below are some interesting ideas for you to consider beyond your walking plan and to challenge yourself further:

Try to walk 15,000 steps per day:

If you feel you need to take it to the next level and 10,000 steps per day is something you can do with no problem at all, aim for 15,000 steps per day. This will be around 7.5 miles instead of the 5 miles for the 10,000 steps distance. Be aware of the additional time and distance involved and plan accordingly. You'd have to spend 33% more time than before if you want to accomplish this rather challenging goal. At this point it becomes interesting looking at other sports and activities options if you are also able to stick to the 15,000 steps per day challenge.

A couple of useful exercises to strengthen your feet:

If your feet or toes start to hurt as you start building up your number of steps and distance of your walks, consider these two exercises as a way to make your feet and toes stronger:

Pulling a towel on the floor with your toes: Sit on a chair and place a small towel flat on the floor or carpet in front of you, with your toes only and without lifting your feet, start pulling the towel towards you, pull the towel with your toes for 12-15 times, rest for about 30 seconds and repeat 2 more times. Total workout is 3 series of 12-15 repetitions each. Do this at least twice a day.

Stand up toe lifts: Stand up on the carpet or with your feet together. Keeping your feet on the floor/carpet, lift your toes only in a slow controlled way for 12-15 times, rest 30 seconds and repeat 2 more times. Do a total of 3 Series of 12-15 repetitions. Do this at least twice a day.

*For an extra bonus** try this exercise with your heels together but your feet open in front of you. Also try with your heels open and your feet closed in front of you. You should feel your chins and calf muscles working differently when you try with the variations of this exercise.

Mix it up - Practice other sports or activities:

If walking 10,000 steps per day is fun but no longer enough, consider mixing up your walks with some jogging or running. Depending on how fit you are or how challenging you want this to be, I've read interesting plans to mix you walks with some jogging/running by an author named Jeff Galloway. In fact I used his plan to train for my first half marathon some years back. He is very understanding of how starting easy to prevent injuries and keep you motivated can work great for you. You can start by walking 10 minutes, then run for 5-10 minutes at a comfortable pace (a pace you can keep a conversation going while running), and end with another 10 minutes' walk. Initially keep your total combined time to 30 minutes, and add 5-10 minutes combined total time during the second week, another 5-10 minutes the third week and so on. Jeff Galloway also has interesting walking/running combination plans for people just getting started into jogging or running. He covers distances from 5K (3.1 miles) and up to the marathon (26.2 miles). I highly recommend you to go online or purchase a book by him if you want to challenge yourself beyond a walking plan.

In addition to walking and running, swimming is an excellent sport. Swimming is a very low impact and very complete sport. Since water acts as a shock absorbent, you can use it to rest your ankles, knees and hips if you at one point injure yourself or get sore on your long walks or runs. Your local YMCA or community pool is a good way to get you started with swimming.

Other very useful sports are cycling and weight lifting. If you live in an area where you can bike safely outdoors, go for it. Cycling is also a very low impact activity and you can enjoy with family and friends. I personally use the stationary bike at the gym for convenience. Most stationary bikes let you customize your level of effort during your workout, plus it's a great to get started if you eventually want to get serious about cycling. Weight lifting is useful to get your body toned if you opt to go with high repetitions with light weight (12-15 or more repetitions per exercise). Getting some strength will also help you with any other activity/sport like long walks, running or cycling. Don't forget also to work your core body (abs, lower back and hips). Having a strong core and good overall body strength can help with preventing injuries from other sports.

The elliptical machine (or similar) at your local gym is great as full body cardio workout. I do use elliptical machine from time, it not only works your legs and hips, but also your arms and shoulders. It's a great cardio workout to add variety to your walking and running. You burn a great deal of calories and it offers a fairly low impact to prevent or heal from injuries. I highly recommend varying the type of exercise or physical activity you practice, even if you have one as your day to day that you prefer. Adding other activities or sports not only refreshes your mind by going to different places, it's fun and if you are rather serious about physical activity, it's one of the best ways to prevent injuries and get all around physically fitter.

Conclusion:

To conclude, I'd like to mention that a walking or any other workout or exercise plan should be seen as part of a holistic approach towards health. In other words, even though this book had in mind getting your motivated and working towards your goal of 10,000 steps per day walk plan, you want to consider all other health important elements like healthy eating habits, getting enough good quality sleep and your family and friends support towards leaving a healthier and fuller life.

I'm currently writing other books about how to prevent and heal from inflammation, healthy plant-based recipes, plant-based smoothies and health topics in general. These upcoming books will be based on my experience with endurance sport and years of reading and experimenting with diets, different type of foods and looking to live a healthy life in general. I hope to see you soon to share this great useful information.

Finally, if you enjoyed this book, please take a moment to share your thoughts by posting an honest review on Amazon. I will greatly appreciate it.

To your healthy living!

BOOK DESCRIPTION:

This book contains useful information on the exercise of walking and how you can benefit from getting into a daily habit of long walks. You'd learn with some guidance the basic elements needed to make your walking plan a success.

Here you'll learn how to get the right mindset and motivation, how to choose the best places to walk and how to setup a successful walking schedule.

You'll also learn the basic gear (minimal) needed to get yourself started with walking every day and start enjoying a healthier and happier lifestyle. In addition you'll get advice for you to be able to tell if your walking plan is working or needs any adjustments. Lastly you'll find out about options available beyond walking 10,000 steps per day and new challenges.

What you will learn:

- How to assess your current fitness and overall wellness levels

- Why you should chose walking as an excellent exercise to improve your health and fitness

- What are the requirements (minimal by the way) to get started with a walking plan

- A detailed step by step plan towards walking 10,000 steps every day

- How to measure the results of a successful walking plan

- What to do once you accomplish your goal of walking 10,000 per day or more

www.ingramcontent.com/pod-product-compliance
Lightning Source LLC
Chambersburg PA
CBHW071310280526
45788CB00004B/1877